Improving Your A1C: Weight Management

Improving A1C: Weight Loss

Improving Your A1C: Weight Management

Pat White

Improving A1C: Weight Loss

Contents

Improving A1C: Weight Loss

Introduction

If eating is likened to driving a car, you will not drive a car with a blindfold. Yet, this is exactly how people go about their meals.

Before you drive, you must learn the road signs, driving etiquette, have experience and a whole lot of other variables.

A driver instinctively knows when to apply the brakes. A lot of people do not know when to apply the brakes when it comes to how much calories they are allowed in a day.

Indeed, a lot of people don't even know when they must stop eating or apply the brakes on a dieting "superhighway."

One of the few brakes at your disposal is:

Exercise. There is a whole body of study—exercise science—which is the systemic study of the mechanisms underlying human movement exercise and physical activity.

Exercise is just one of the brakes for eating run amok. Who needs some form of exercise most? We all need exercise.

Exercise is any bodily activity that enables an

individual to maintain physical fitness. Exercise enhances overall health and wellness. When engaged in frequently, it helps in preventing aging, strengthening muscles, increasing growth and strengthening the cardiovascular system.

Some other reasons you must engage in exercise is to hone athletic skills, to manage your weight and simply for fun and or as an occupation.

With food and dieting, it is important to have a plan when you will eat each meal and stick with that plan. It is equally important to change your behaviors around food if you have not already done so.

This is because many people have habits that make weight loss very difficult.

Overeating, which is one of those behaviors can lead to weight gaining and often obesity.

Overeating is the excess food consumed in a given time in relation to the energy that organism expends.

If you do not make room for a calorie deficit if you are obese, your chance of weight loss is nearly impossible. A calorie deficit is where you do not consume all your daily calorie budget.

If I were talking about money, it would be a surplus—a sort of savings which is a good management of public or personal finance.

For food, it is a good range—a deficit—which will enable your body to tap into the accumulated fat thereby resulting in weight loss. A calorie deficit is the difference between the amount of energy you eat and expend—the shortfall of energy as a result of consuming less than your daily budget.

Engaging in extended body activity will help burn off excess fat.

If your body calls for 2000 daily calorie budget and you consume only 1500 calories, you have obviously denied your body 500 calories. But the body knows where to make up this deficit. The body taps into the accumulated fat in your body and collects that 500 calories.

If you continue on this part of having a calorie deficit, over time, you start to lose weight.

To calculate a calorie deficit is simple. It goes like this. If you eat more than your body requires and your activities can burn, you accumulate fat and so gains weight. However, if you burn more calories than you eat, you lose weight.

Let's stop for a moment and look at the last sentence. That sentence says you can eat as much as you can.

The question most people will not ask themselves is: Can I burn more than I ate? This is the question we must answer. This is the nervous system of your weight loss. Any weight loss.

The only pieces of information you need to succeed in weight loss are those dealing with: Knowing the number of calories you consume and burn daily. It is that simple.

Knowing the number of calories you consume is somewhat

straightforward if you learn and master it but knowing the amounts of calories you burn is hard. This is where this book comes in handy.

Chapter Two: Importance of light exercise—Walking

Before you engage in any serious exercise please consult your doctor. Walking is perhaps one of the most convenient exercises we engage in without really giving it a second thought.

Walking is effective. It is so effective that when you engage in it at least 1 hour 3 times a week, you start to feel good in no time.

Walking is the most underrated form of exercise. It is the ideal type of exercise when you are just getting started with exercises.

Walking is just as good as running. However, you will do much more walking to reap the same benefits as you would running.

Walking slowly in a park over a period of 30 or more minutes will enable you reduce the risk of high blood pressure, high cholesterol and diabetes.

When you walk for exercise, it is recommended that you walk at least 4.5 miles at a brisk pace. Put differently, you would have walked 1hour 18 minutes briskly to cover

4.5 miles. A runner would have achieved the same benefit by running 38 minutes—3miles. However, running is not for everybody.

Different exercises in general helps you burn calories. When the same total energy is used for a brisk intensity walking as for vigorous-intensity running, it will yield the same reductions in high cholesterol and diabetes. The risks in high blood pressure and coronary heart disease will be reduced too.

Think of exercise—walking—in the same light as vehicular brakes. A brake serves the function of stopping a moving vehicle. Exercises serve as a brake in stopping you from the risks of various diseases like coronary heart diseases, diabetes and many others.

There are many reasons you should engage in some type of exercise regularly. Apart from weight management, some other reasons are listed below extolling the benefits for exercise:

A.   Helps to build your aerobic power. Your aerobic capacity is the body's ability to work at maximum capacity by getting oxygen and distributing it to your body effortlessly. You may want to know that we are likely to lose about 1% efficiency of aerobic capacity every year. If you are 40 and lose such efficiency every year, by the time you are 50 you may have lost 10%

of your aerobic power. It is down hill from there. Perhaps, you may have heard of some breathing problems people experience from time to time. By age 70, it is estimated that 30% of our aerobic power must have been lost. That is a lot of aerobic power lost and you can imagine what such loss does to the body. We can cut the loss by half with exercises. I want you to picture the man or woman with their tank of oxygen and all that rubber tubes carried or dragged along to everywhere they travel on a daily basis. I make that video image to show how important it is to strengthen and maintain your aerobic power. It is very important. Walking regularly can build your aerobic capacity.

B.   Builds your immune power. Your immune power is what protects you from infection. Some people are easily infected with minor diseases. Some people too can get cured of diseases in 3 days while others may last 3 weeks before they get cured. Your immune system plays an important role maintaining a healthy response to stress. The stress hormone—cortisol—is a health enemy number one. Scientists have warned for years that elevated levels of cortisol will lower immune function and bone density, increase weight gain, elevate cholesterol and blood pressure; and cause heart diseases. Chronic stress and elevated cortisol levels will ultimately lead to increased risk for depression and lower life expectancy. A simple regular walk in the park will reduce all these. This is why exercise is very important for you. Regular exercise can reverse some of the deleterious effect of aging.

C.   Builds muscle mass. Exercise help you to build muscle mass. If you don't engage in exercises, you will lose about 1% of your muscle strength every year. While walking and running will help you maintain your muscle strength, the best exercise to build muscle mass is weight lifting for fitness. The loss of muscle mass/tissue is a natural part of aging. Hopefully, we will age but aging must not be painful and ugly. Walking helps you age gracefully.

D.	Walking enable you to reduce blood pressure. High blood pressure is the number one form of heart disease. When we do not eat right, plaque build up in the arteries becomes inevitable resulting from high-fat diets. However, exercise helps you fight back the plaque build-up. As you attack the plaque with regular exercises, your blood flow becomes better and therefore reduces the blood pressure. Simultaneously, hypertension decreases because regular exercises strengthens the heart which is also a muscle. The stronger the heart (muscle) is the better it pumps blood efficiently through your arteries.

E.   Lower your risk of type 2 diabetes. Type 2 diabetes is on a rampage at this time. It is known that the higher your BMI, the higher your risk for heart diseases like high blood pressure, type

2 diabetes etc. You may succumb to gallstones, apnea and other breathing problems. There are literatures that estimate that over 7 million deaths worldwide will be as a result of heart disease. It is estimated that by the year 2031—a little over a decade from now—over 336 million people

worldwide will be diabetic. The best weapon against this threat is exercise. Exercise can ward off the advancement because your body's ability to metabolize glucose would have been improved tremendously. You can also help your glucose/sugar level by discriminating on food types that you consume.

F. Walking exercise helps reduce body fat. Are you obese or overweight? Your body mass index (BMI) will answer this question for you. If you are on the high end of the BMI, walking or running will help your muscle burn body fat fast. If you are in the habit of spending more than the allowed calorie budget, you should increase the daily frequency of walking. If you walked 3x a week for one hour daily, perhaps you need to double it if you truly want to see any noticeable effect. On the other hand, you may be better off cutting down on the calories.

G.   Your breathing will be improved.

H.   Boosts your energy

I. Your sex drive will improve. When we exercise—walking or running—regularly, it enables the endocrine glands to produce adequate hormones and more muscle mass.

Enough hormones and muscle mass are the road to greater stimulation to produce androgens. Androgens are the group of sex hormones that give men their "lion" male characteristics. It's the hormone that puts the "tiger" in females too. This hormone which is enhanced because of exercises enable a better sex function and keeps you fit and Eveready.

J. Lowers risk of depression. Your mood improves as your outlook on life becomes warmer if it were cold earlier. Every situation is not all about popping one pill or another. Some of our psychological disorders are better helped with simple exercises than behavioral treatments. Most medicines have their side effects. The only side effect of yoga, walking or running are few muscle aches in the early days of adjusting to the new activities. With regular exercises, you lower your risk of depression because exercises cause your body to release endorphins. Endorphins are the naturally occurring feel good neurotransmitters. Endorphins do not take long to kick in during your exercises. You feel good and less likely to waste your time on depression inducing thoughts.

K.   Builds cognitive functioning. The overall impacts of regular exercises on your overall systems are the improvements in your cognitive functioning. Walking is not a tedious exercise. The same could be said of yoga. Even in their simplicity, regular exercise helps your neuron stay in shape particularly in the memory areas of your brain. Regular walking can help the hippocampus—brain's memory area—function efficiently with health and vitality. Regular exercise benefits the brain memory area in the lowering of cortisol. Remember that high levels of cortisol increase the risk of stress and ultimately depression.

L. Exercise boosts Intelligence. You think fast. You think outside the box and on your feet. As your memory improves so does your intellectual capacity. This is because as oxygen flows efficiently to your systems especially your brain not only does your hippocampus benefit but that part of the brain charged with reasoning and planning (prefrontal cortex) even performs faster and more efficiently too. Oh, what about the risk of dementia?

M.   Yes. Exercise lowers the risk of dementia. So far,

you may have
noticed the many
impact of exercise
on our systems
especially on the
heart and the brain.
There are more.
Exercise is free
candy in the store.
Be a child again and
partake of this candy
for as long as you
want and take all the
quantity you want.
Exercise lowers your
chances for

dementia. Such dementia may be the result of a cardiovascular illness. But since you exercise your risk of coronary diseases is reduced because of improved blood flow and so also are those coronary diseases that lead to dementia. You will recall reading that by improving the blood flow to your brain, you will preserve the neurons in your brain. The preservation of the neurons is an added advantage if you eventually develop the disease. This is because exercise slows the disease—Alzheimer's—down. You will notice that some of the coronary diseases and diabetes are the epicenter to many inefficiencies in our body systems.

N. Good & Satisfying sleep. When you regularly exercise (walking, yoga etc.), you experience the excellent benefits of sleep. There's a substantial body of scientific evidence that exercise improves sleep.

When you exercise regularly as a routine, it can contribute to a healthier, more restful relaxation.

Exercise may help alleviate sleep issues such as insomnia. Sleeping better also improves your immune functioning and can even lower the risk for heart disease and cognitive impairment.

With all the above benefits of simple, mild and soothing exercise of walking, would you rather leave these benefits to others to enjoy and live longer healthier lives?

There should be no flimsy excuse not to claim the benefits of this light walking workout of one-hour

3x a week or 30mins daily.

If you do not have a walking sneaker, perhaps you are now itching to go get one. Or perhaps you need one more reason.

Walking reduces the risk of arthritis. Arthritis causes pain and fatigue and may become a regular part of your day. It is extremely painful and may disfigure your fine body shape. The disease can be so debilitating that holding a cup of coffee becomes seriously tasking.

Over time, those kinds of symptoms can make the sufferer feel frustrated, anxious, angry and sometimes, depressed. It gets to a stage where the sufferer might neither be able to dress themselves nor able to do anything for themselves.

Middle-aged and older adults suffer the effects of the varying kinds of this disease. Arthritis occurs mostly within these age ranges because we get old there are abnormalities in the cartilage and outgrowth of bones in the joints.

Walking, yoga and Tai Chi are soft and mild exercises that can reduce the effects of arthritis.

Running and other more physical type exercises are not recommended as such exercises may exacerbate the already bad situation.

As with any exercise, consult a doctor before you start one.

How does exercise work for weight management? Actually, it is quite simple.

Your body calls for a certain number of calories. That would be your daily calorie budget. This is calculated based on your present weight, height (BMI).

You may want to read my book *Weight Loss: Eat Well, Eat Clean, Eat Right.*

Depending on your present BMI, you may want to manage your weight: Weight gain or weight loss or maintain your weight as is.

By walking or running, you can eat what you want and as much as you like however, the extent of your exercises could be longer or shorter. It depends on how much you eat and how much weight you have decided to lose or gain.

One key word in food consumption is moderation. One other keyword in food intake is calories. Your body uses calories from food for thinking, walking, running, breathing and other important activities.

If your daily calorie budget calls for 3000 calories and you decide on a calorie deficit of 500 calories, you just placed yourself on a restricted diet.

This is not the same as fasting. If you maintain this calorie deficit, you will still achieve ketosis—burning fat instead of sugar—

without all the headaches that comes with the attempt to be a big loser.

Placing yourself on a restricted diet is just one way to attain your BMI and therefore an optimum level.

If your BMI tells you to adjust and if your daily calorie budget calls for 3000 calories and you decide on maintaining this calorie budget even while you know you are obese because your BMI tells you so, you must lose weight.

Since, you love your food so much so, that you abhor anything that suggests a restricted diet, you must find another way to optimal health.

The other available way is to burn excess fat through walking exercise. If you walk constantly and maintain your calorie budget, you will still achieve ketosis—burning fat instead of sugar—without all the headaches that comes with the attempt to be a big loser.

Walking is a great form of physical activity and it is free. It is also low risk and you can engage in it even in your room. Since we need energy—calories—to enable all the complex chemical reactions that allow us to breathe, move from place to place, think and function normally, our calorie needs vary from person to person.

Calorie needs are also affected by our weight, genes, sex and especially our activity level. We know that we need to burn more calories than we consume in order to lose weight.

One way to burn excess fat is to keep walking. If your daily calorie budget calls for 3000 and you go over that budget, you can remedy the deficit by burning the excess calories through brisk walk.

For a 130-pound individual, walking briskly at a pace of 3.5 mph burns 80 to 90 calories per half-hour.

For an hour at same pace, you will burn 160 to 180 calories. For a 200-pound person, a 3.5 mph pace burns about 120 calories per half-hour or 240 calories per hour.

Take a look at how much calories you can burn per an hour of walking exercise and consider if this is too little or too much to burn per walk-out.

A rule of thumb is that about approximately 100 calories per mile are burned for a 180-pound individual and 65 calories per mile are burned for a 120-pound person.

Your weight and the distance you walk are the two most important factors in how much calories you burn during a walking exercise. Perhaps at this point it will be a good idea to make a list of various foods and how much calories they contain.

This will give you an idea of how much calories you consume and better yet, how much workout you need to put in to lose excess pounds.

Chapter Three: Calories in Various Foods

Let's start with America's go to foods (fast food).

Burger King:

Whoppers	Calories	Sodium (mg)	Carbs(g)	Sugar (g)
Whopper	660	980	49	11
Whopper w/chees e	740	1340	50	11
Bacon Cheese whooper	790	1560	50	11
Double Whoppe	900	1050	49	11

r				
Dbl. with cheese	980	1410	50	11
Triple Whoppe r	1220	1470	50	11
Bacon King	1150	2150	49	10
Large French Fry	430	640	60	0
Ultimate Breakfast Platter	1230	2550	122	33
Sausage, Egg & Cheese Croissan' wich	520	910	30	4
Hash Browns (small)	250	410	24	0
Coca Cola Classic	380		102	
Sprite (Lg)	380		102	

McDonald's:

Menu Item	Sodium(mg)	Calories	Carbs(g)	Sugars(g)
Big Mac	950	540	45	9
McRib	870	480	45	12
Big N' Tasty	720	460	37	8
Angus Bacon & Cheese	2070	790	63	13
Angus Deluxe	1700	750	61	10
Filet-O-Fish	640	380	38	5
McChicken	600	360	40	5
Single Bacon Smokehouse Burger	1580	840	62	18
Dbl. Bacon Smokehouse Burger	1920	1130	63	18
French Fries (Lg)	350	510	66	0

Coca Cola Classic (Lg)	70	290	77	77
Diet Coke (Lg)	95	0	0	0
Sprite (Lg)		310	83	83
Sausage McMuffin with Egg	920	450	30	2
Bacon, Egg & Cheese Biscuit	1160	420	37	3
Big Breakfast	1560	740	51	3

Other Regular Foods

Food Item	plain	Calories after Dressing added (1)	Calories after dressing added (2)	Calories after dressings added (3)	Added (4)
Bagel (3.5oz)	270	With butter 300-350	Cream cheese 320-367	With eggs 295-330	With eggs, cheese & bacon 672
2 slices of white bread	132	With butter approx. 178	With cream cheese 229-280	With eggs 157-187	With eggs, cheese & bacon 225-281
Slice of Pizza	266	Cheese Pizza Approx... 291	Pepperoni Pizza Approx. 300	Sausage Pizza Approx. 280	New York Pizza Approx. 680
Coffee	12(oz) black 4	16 (oz) with 2tbsp cream & 2tsp sugar 74	12 (oz) with 2 tbsp cream & 1tsp sugar 72	16 (oz) with 2 Splenda & cream 35	--
Tea	8oz 2	With 1 tsp of sugar 17	With 2 tsp 32	With 2 tsp & 2 tbsp 50	
Whopper					
Baked potato	163	With butter 1 tbsp 263	With butter & Sour Cream	Medium baked potato with	Medium baked potato With 2

			313	Salsa 190	oz Tuna and a dab of Mayo 275
Large fries	1 serving of baked French fry 130-140	1 serving of French fry 156	Medium Fries 340-380-410	Large French fries 430-510-530 Fast Food joints	

- Some calorie count in the chart above are estimates.

- 1 serving of French fries equals 156 calories or 3 oz or 10 pieces of French fries.

There are important reasons for the illustrations above. The charts are intended to guide our eating choices.

There are many factors that drive our eating habits among which are emotion, taste, culture, marketing and advertising, economic status and most importantly, health and fitness.

The purpose of this book is health and fitness through your eating habits. An overweight or obese person whose desire is to lose weight will under the circumstances choose differently than a skinny underweight person.

This is so because a person whose metabolism/activity allows them to eat whatever they want has no concerns of weight gain.

Though taste is a major factor in our decisions, it often comes second to the caloric values and fat contents of the food items.

For obese individual whose decision is mostly driven by weight loss, caloric values and fat contents are at the top of their minds.

For example, your decision might be influenced by how much you weigh now. If you are overweight or obese, you are likely to reduce your calorie budget.

If one was to make a breakfast decision from the charts above based on a 2100 daily calorie budget, it is likely that the decision is unlikely to budget over 700 calories for breakfast alone.

If the decision-maker plans to leave room for snacks later in the day, the caloric values must be considered in the total daily calorie budget.

So, if I decide to go to one of the fast food joints above, the best I can do for choices is very limited. For example, if I choose BK's Croissan'wich =520 calories. I cannot afford to add a small bag of hash browns because that will make me go over the budget.

I cannot even eye the Ultimate Breakfast Platter that is worth 1230 calories.

The only way out is to eat half the meal in a proportionality to allow for only 615 calories, half of 1230. But, is that not a waste of food and money? However, one can choose the

Croissan'wich and a cup of coffee and you will still meet what your daily calorie count calls for.

You may as well consider McDonald's Big breakfast with medium biscuit =740 calories. If you must add a 16 oz cup of coffee with Splenda, you only exceeded your calorie budget by 44. You are likely to burn more than 44 calories if you walk more than 10 minutes back home.

Overindulgence in fast food joints daily is not encouraged. However, that does not eliminate it entirely from your choices.

Indulging in your favorite fast food should be a choice only 20% of the time.

This is because eating what you love is part of happiness. If you are not happy with your diet regimen, you may not succeed in weight management because you will get frustrated and fail.

Sometimes, you try again and fail again. You are unintentionally doing a yo-yo diet which is not good for the body. There are many studies that claim that yo-yo dieting can increase the risk of diabetes.

This is because the constant changes of your body weight reflect the problems inside your body.

Blood sugar highs are always dangerous and fluctuations in weight can make them worse.

The purpose is not to punish but to reward you to succeed. The purpose is to enable you create a habit that will eventually help you to achieve the healthy weight and to find a way of eating that you can sustain for as long as you live.

Most people in the food industry will tell you that if you want your food exactly how you want it, cook it yourself. That way, you know exactly what the inputs are and therefore you can predict the outcome.

If you want to predict what is exactly in your

meal without cooking it yourself, you can also do that with nearly a precise accuracy.

Let us consider another breakfast. A bagel with the works and a cup of coffee. You'd be surprised that the outcome of calories based on this simple choice could be very enormous.

Even if you like drinking your tea with milk, cream, or sugar, you don't need to obsess over the small amount of calories in it. The cup of tea contributes a negligible amount of calories, and if you are adding only a teaspoon or a cube of sugar, the contribution of a few calories from the sugar is not worth worrying about.

The good practice of counting calories and being overly obsessive over the nutritional details of each food can itself become more destructive than too many calories themselves.

There are many ways calorie counting can become overly obsessive. Being overly obsessive of calorie counting can lead to eating disorder.

Counting calories in itself should not be looked upon as a bad habit. Like everything else, too much of engaging in it, is bad. You and I, knows that calories are a source for the body's natural energy source from the diet. A bottle of water is healthy so also is a cup of tea. Even sweetened tea is healthy. Sweetened tea can be part of a healthy diet and lifestyle.

Chapter Four: Creating Daily Calorie Deficits

Being on the track to creating calorie deficits daily for as long as it takes to meet your weight goal is tough yet very easy.

If you want to plan anything, you need information. You need to set goals. You need benchmarks no matter what subjects you are dealing with. You need to understand what you are about to step into. Creating a heathy you, requires you to understand a couple of a few simple things. To not understand and practice these few criteria is simply a creation of a failing weight loss strategy or a weight gaining strategy.

You need to understand how to create a calorie deficit scenario. You need to understand what calorie deficit is, what calorie budget is, and when to lose or gain weight.

You need to understand how to monitor your calories intake. You need to understand how to make smart food choices. It is your life. Your life depends on it.

Your choices (minus other variables) determine a short life and longevity. Creating a calorie deficit is very essential for your weight loss.

Below are some more tips on how to achieve and sustain calorie deficit and therefore a sustained weight loss.

1. Establish your BMI. Then create your basal metabolic rate (your

BMR). Your BMR is the calories your body needs to maintain its current weight at rest. Consider your age, sex, height and weight.

Better still, find how many calories your BMI calls for and budget your calories to work towards what your BMI called for. Remember, if you are seriously obese, you must slowly work towards what your BMI called for. Do not just dive into it. Better still, consult a dietician if your situation is dire.

2.

Calculate your total daily energy expenditure. This expenditure accounts for your daily activity level. Your daily activity determines how much calorie your body burns daily if such activity remained constant. Multiply your BMR by your activity level or factor (a) minimal or no exercise at all: BMR * 1.2

(b) Lightly active—2 days/week: BMR * 1.375

(c) Moderately active—4days a week: BMR * 1.55

(d)Very active—6days/week: BMR *1.725

(f)Very, Very active (very hard exercise, hard work and sports: BMR *1.9

Having done the above, you can aim for gradual weight loss.

3. Set the Weight Loss Goal: The weight loss should be gradual— about one pound a week is very good. Set a calorie deficit to adhere to. What about 500 calorie deficit a day? That comes to 3,500 calories a week. That will be a good point to start.

4. Monitor your food/calorie consumption. Be mindful of food portions. Be mindful not to overindulge. Choose whole foods like fruits, lean proteins and vegetables. While choosing salads, be mindful of the dressings, snacks and sauces; they pack a punch too in calories.

5. If possible, increase your level of physical activities like walking and finally, be patient as the weight will sooner or later start to fall off as you stay consistent and persistent in following the guidelines.

Chapter Five: How Many Calories to Consume a Day to Lose Weight.

Losing the weight is hard yet doable. When it comes to losing the weight, it boils down to calories, calories and calories. The number of calories you can eat per day depends on many factors like your age, gender, size and very importantly your activity level. You should follow what your BMI calls for. Establish your BMR as earlier discussed in the last chapter. If you are a woman the general recommendations are as follows:

Age: 19-30; Calorie requirement: 1800—2400

Age: 31-60; Calorie requirement: 1600—2200

Age: 61- above; aim for 1600—2000; the older we get, the less activities we engage in hence the less calories requirement.

Men:

When it comes to men the calorie requirement differs. The recommended daily calorie intake for an adult man in the United

States varies based on factors we listed earlier also for women. Various countries have their recommendations for daily calorie intake. For this exercise however, we are using the statistics of the USA.

According to the recent dietary guidelines (2020-2025) for Americans, the calorie recommendation for adult men is 2200-3200. However, this is not one size fits all. Remember your BMI (Body Mass Index) & your BMR (Basal Metabolic Rate) are different from other individuals. So, design your calorie intake just for you.

These estimates are just general guidelines that won't apply to everyone. Design your personal calorie deficit to assist your weight loss goals.

Always have it at the back of your mind that weight loss is just about reduced intake of calories, it is also about intake of the right nutrients. The give and take between the reduced intake of excess calories and the intake of the right nutrients is essential for a long-term success.

Chapter Six: Okra

If your attempts at losing weight is hard, don't sweat it. Okra could be your best go to solution while doing all the other things you were already doing when it comes to losing weight.

If you already developed diabetes, okra could help you too. I know people who share a love hate relationship with okra.

They say the sliminess is what they dislike.

Well, when you suffer diabetes resulting from obesity, the sliminess is better than the effects of all the drugs one takes to reduce the impact of diabetes-related illnesses.

Commonly known as Lady Finger, okra can be used raw in salads. The leaves can also be used in salads. Okra can be cooked and served with a variety of food like rice, yam, and potato among others.

The more times you consume okra in your diet the better for your weight control. But that is not the only ways to prepare okra.

Okra can be specially prepped specifically for weight loss purpose. If your plan is to lose weight through diet modification approach and more importantly if you want to sustain optimal body mass index (BMI) so that excess body fat will not elevate your risk of diabetes, depression, cancer and other health conditions caused by overweight, okra—yes, this simple veggie—could be the sustainer.

Prep for Okra Juice. How to Make Okra Water

It is simple and straightforward.

a. Fill a gallon with clean water. In USA, an empty milk gallon will serve this purpose very well.
b. Select 10-12 finger long okra. Wash the Lady Fingers properly under

running water.
Remove the ends of
the okra and slice
them in half
longitudinally from
end to end.

c. Put the slices in the
gallon of water.

d. Let it sit overnight—
twenty-four hours—
while stored in the
refrigerator as the
slimy sap seeps into
the water.

e. Drink it—a full
glass—first thing in

the morning with an empty stomach.

f. Continue to drink the juice, first thing in the morning on an empty stomach every morning until the gallon is empty but not after 7 days from the same gallon.

You may want to take out the pods and squeeze out the sap

with your hands for the last drink from this prep.

g. After 7 days, pour the leftover okra juice/water out, wash the gallon clean, sanitize and prepare afresh, juice with fresh okra pods and water.

If you make this a longtime plan and follow

up on it, you will reap the benefits.

You will be amazed at the result you get. If you are diabetic, you will start to achieve better and improved A1C results without all the hassles you were used to.

You will also notice a steady decline in your pounds. The benefits of okra juice are many. Let us look at a few.

1. Perhaps, the most important benefit is that Okra stabilizes your body's sugar levels.
2. Okra juice helps you fight against anemia.
3. Okra juice helps prevent, control diabetes.
4. Okra juice lowers cholesterol level
5. Okra juice is a very good body cleanser.
6. Drinking Okra juice helps keep the

intestinal tract functioning as naturally required.

7. Drinking the Okra juice helps in bettering the immune system

8. Drinking Okra water reduces asthma attack.

9. Regular consumption of Okra juice improves skin health.

10. And for the 10th benefit, Okra juice

helps strengthen our bones. Most of us expect to get old. And when we do, we desire strong bones. The folate found in Okra helps in increasing the density of the bones and prevents bone related illnesses like osteoporosis and of course arthritis.

If you deem slimy okra juice undrinkable, there

are other ways to prep the okra pods.

The pharaohs of Egypt whose staple among many, is okra, gets their okra prepared in various other ways. They fry the pods. They boiled the okra with salt added. They add cut okra pods in soups and in stews.

The leaves are also eaten in various ways. Our grandparents are food scientists if you must know. Cooking a soup with okra is a culture practiced especially in Africa and exported to all the areas you can find black folks.

Chapter Seven: Conclusion

A lot of obese people make one big mistake. They have a need to lose the weight and when they develop the desire and hunger to lose the weight, they lose interest one month into the regimen. We forget that all the weight was gained not in one month but over the years. It is also going to be months and or years to get to a desired goal.

No overweight person gained all that weight overnight therefore, it will take time albeit slowly. Slow progress is a progress. Never underrate slow progress. Do not rush it. Do it according to plan spread over time. Take it one step at a time. Perhaps, your first step could be substituting whole milk with 2% milk. Or it could be replacing white bread with whole wheat bread. It can be replacing your soda with diet variety or simply water thereby eliminating high levels of sugar. It does not matter how small you start but start somewhere.

Record your progress no matter how slow you

might assume it is progressing

Look for Support:

In whatever we do especially attempts to lose weight can be helped and reinforced when you have support.